THIS PLANNER
Belongs To:

I'm PREGNANT!

DUE DATE

How I found out

My reaction

WHAT I AM MOST EXCITED ABOUT

WHO I TOLD FIRST

WHAT I WANT YOU TO KNOW

MY BIRTH PLAN *Ideas*

WHO I WANT IN THE DELIVERY ROOM:

TYPE OF BIRTH

☐ **VAGINAL**   ☐ **WATER BIRTH**

☐ **C-SECTION**   ☐ **VBAC**

THOUGHTS ABOUT BIRTH AND WHAT IS MOST IMPORTANT TO ME

GETTING READY FOR THE BIG DAY: TO DO

NOTES & IDEAS (lighting, music, etc.)

40 Weeks

PREGNANCY *Tracker*

♥♥♥♥♥♥♥♥♥♥♥♥♥♥♥♥♥♥♥♥♥

Keep track of how you're feeling every week of your pregnancy.

APPOINTMENT *Tracker*

Keep track of your pre-natal classes and doctor appointments.

DATE	TIME	ADDRESS	PURPOSE

BABY SHOPPING *List*

Start planning for the arrival of your baby by using the shopping list below.

Undershirts	Crib	Bottles
Socks	Bassinet	Bottle Liners
Pajamas	Baby Bath tub	Nursing Bra & Pads
Sweaters	Car Seat	Breast Pump
Onesies	Stroller	Formula
Hats	High Chair	Pacifiers
Bibs	Play Pen	Bottle Brush
Blanket	Baby Swing	Burp Cloths
Diaper Bag	Monitor	Bottle Sanitizer
Mitts	Change Table	Nipples
Diapers	Rocking Chair	Baby Powder
Booties	Night Light	Baby Wipes
Receiving Blankets	Mobile	
Crib Sheet	Bouncer	
Wash Cloths	Nail Clippers	
Towels	Teething Toys	
	Baby Wipes	
	Diaper Pail	

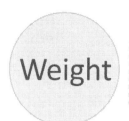 Weight

PREGNANCY *Tracker*

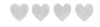 *Weight Tracker Chart*

It's important to keep track of your weight throughout your pregnancy.
Record your weight in the chart below every week, starting at week 4.

WEEKLY WEIGHT TRACKER

4		12		20		28		36	
5		13		21		29		37	
6		14		22		30		38	
7		15		23		31		39	
8		16		24		32		40	
9		17		25		33			
10		18		26		34			
11		19		27		35			

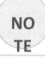 **NOTE** According to the American Pregnancy Association, pregnant women should consume up to 300 more calories a day. Further, healthy eating is critical to your baby's development which means you should make sure to maintain a well-balanced diet, high in nutrients and proteins.

HEALTHY FOOD *Ideas*

VEGETABLES & LOW SUGAR FRUIT	PROTEINS	COMPLEX CARBS	HEALTHY FATS	SUPPLEMENTS
Leafy greens (spinach, etc.)	Organic meat	Beets	Avocado	Vitamin D
Broccoli	Liver	Carrots	Olive Oil	Fish Oil
Cauliflower	Bone Broth	Sweet Potatoes	Coconut Oil	Algae Oil
Cabbage	Beans	Yams	Yogurt	Probiotics
Asparagus	Lentils	Parsnips	Almonds	Ginger Pills
Cucumber	Flax Seed	Turnips	Mixed Nuts	Licorice Root
Mushrooms	Pumpkin Seed	Pumpkin	Soybean	Magnesium
Celery	Chia Seed	Buckwheat	Olives	Krill Oil
Radish	Salmon	Brown Rice	Nut butter	Iron Pills
Grapefruit & Melon	Herring	Squash		
Berries (all kinds)				
Peaches (with skin)				

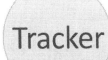

Tracker

PRE-NATAL *Visits*

♥♥♥♥♥ *Important Dates* ♥♥♥♥♥

Keep track of your pre-natal appointments and include a summary of each visit.

		Summary of Appointment
Date		
How far along?		
Your Weight		
Blood Pressure		
Fetal Heart Rate		
Doctor		

NOTES:

Next Appointment.:

		Summary of Appointment
Date		
How far along?		
Your Weight		
Blood Pressure		
Fetal Heart Rate		
Doctor		

NOTES:

Next Appointment.:

		Summary of Appointment
Date		
How far along?		
Your Weight		
Blood Pressure		
Fetal Heart Rate		
Doctor		

NOTES:

Next Appointment.:

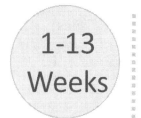

FIRST *Trimester*

1-13 Weeks

Journal your thoughts and feelings during each trimester so you can later reflect on your pregnancy journey.

HOW I FELT DURING MY FIRST TRIMESTER

MY FAVORITE MEMORIES

SYMPTOMS & CRAVINGS

ENERGY

SLEEP

CRAVINGS

MOODS

TO DO LIST: 1st TRIMESTER

FIRST TRIMESTER *Photos*

MEMORIES ARE FOREVER

14-27 Weeks

SECOND *Trimester*

HOW I FELT DURING MY SECOND TRIMESTER

....
....
....
....
....

MY FAVORITE MEMORIES

....
....
....
....

SYMPTOMS & CRAVINGS

....
....
....
....
....
....
....
....
....
....

ENERGY

SLEEP

CRAVINGS

MOODS

TO DO LIST: 2nd TRIMESTER

SECOND TRIMESTER *Photos*

MEMORIES ARE FOREVER

28-40 Weeks

THIRD *Trimester*

HOW I FELT DURING MY THIRD TRIMESTER

MY FAVORITE MEMORIES

SYMPTOMS & CRAVINGS

ENERGY

SLEEP

CRAVINGS

MOODS

TO DO LIST: 3rd TRIMESTER

THIRD TRIMESTER *Photos*

MEMORIES ARE FOREVER

MY BABY *Shower*

BABY SHOWER PHOTOS

GAMES PLAYED

ON THE MENU

HIGHLIGHTS & MEMORIES

MY BABY *Shower Gifts*

Keep track of your baby shower gifts and send thank you notes

NAME	GIFT	ADDRESS	SENT?
			☐
			☐
			☐
			☐
			☐
			☐
			☐
			☐
			☐
			☐
			☐
			☐
			☐
			☐
			☐
			☐

NURSERY *Planner*

| COLOR SCHEME IDEAS: | | | |

ITEM TO PURCHASE	PRICE	NOTES

FURNITURE IDEAS

DECORATIVE IDEAS

BABY NAME *Ideas*

TOP 3 BOY NAMES

NAME MEANINGS

TOP 3 GIRL NAMES

NAME MEANINGS

BABY NAME RESOURCES (LIST YOUR FAVORITE PARENTING & PREGNANCY WEBSITES):

OTHER BOY NAME POSSIBILITIES	OTHER GIRL NAME POSSIBILITES

HOSPITAL *Checklist*

FOR ME	FOR PARTNER	FOR BABY

PREGNANCY SHOPPING *List*

BABY CLOTHING

SUPPLIES/MEDICATION

FURNITURE/TOYS

FIRST TRIMESTER SHOPPING

SECOND TRIMESTER SHOPPING

THIRD TRIMESTER SHOPPING

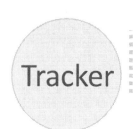

Tracker | FETAL *Movement*

Starting around week 16, keep track of when you feel your baby move.

WEEK 16	TIME	NOTES
MON		
TUE		
WED		
THU		
FRI		
SAT		
SUN		

WEEK 17	TIME	NOTES
MON		
TUE		
WED		
THU		
FRI		
SAT		
SUN		

WEEK 18	TIME	NOTES
MON		
TUE		
WED		
THU		
FRI		
SAT		
SUN		

WEEK 19	TIME	NOTES
MON		
TUE		
WED		
THU		
FRI		
SAT		
SUN		

WEEK 20	TIME	NOTES
MON		
TUE		
WED		
THU		
FRI		
SAT		
SUN		

WEEK 21	TIME	NOTES
MON		
TUE		
WED		
THU		
FRI		
SAT		
SUN		

WEEK 22	TIME	NOTES
MON		
TUE		
WED		
THU		
FRI		
SAT		
SUN		

WEEK 23	TIME	NOTES
MON		
TUE		
WED		
THU		
FRI		
SAT		
SUN		

WEEK 24	TIME	NOTES
MON		
TUE		
WED		
THU		
FRI		
SAT		
SUN		

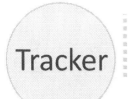

Tracker FETAL *Movement*

WEEK 25	TIME	NOTES
MON		
TUE		
WED		
THU		
FRI		
SAT		
SUN		

WEEK 26	TIME	NOTES
MON		
TUE		
WED		
THU		
FRI		
SAT		
SUN		

WEEK 27	TIME	NOTES
MON		
TUE		
WED		
THU		
FRI		
SAT		
SUN		

WEEK 28	TIME	NOTES
MON		
TUE		
WED		
THU		
FRI		
SAT		
SUN		

WEEK 29	TIME	NOTES
MON		
TUE		
WED		
THU		
FRI		
SAT		
SUN		

WEEK 30	TIME	NOTES
MON		
TUE		
WED		
THU		
FRI		
SAT		
SUN		

WEEK 31	TIME	NOTES
MON		
TUE		
WED		
THU		
FRI		
SAT		
SUN		

WEEK 32	TIME	NOTES
MON		
TUE		
WED		
THU		
FRI		
SAT		
SUN		

WEEK 33	TIME	NOTES
MON		
TUE		
WED		
THU		
FRI		
SAT		
SUN		

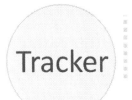

Tracker

FETAL Movement

WEEK 34	TIME	NOTES
MON		
TUE		
WED		
THU		
FRI		
SAT		
SUN		

WEEK 35	TIME	NOTES
MON		
TUE		
WED		
THU		
FRI		
SAT		
SUN		

WEEK 36	TIME	NOTES
MON		
TUE		
WED		
THU		
FRI		
SAT		
SUN		

WEEK 37	TIME	NOTES
MON		
TUE		
WED		
THU		
FRI		
SAT		
SUN		

WEEK 38	TIME	NOTES
MON		
TUE		
WED		
THU		
FRI		
SAT		
SUN		

WEEK 39	TIME	NOTES
MON		
TUE		
WED		
THU		
FRI		
SAT		
SUN		

WEEK 40	TIME	NOTES
MON		
TUE		
WED		
THU		
FRI		
SAT		
SUN		

NOTES		

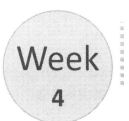

Week 4

PREGNANCY *Journal*

Your baby is the size of a poppy seed!

TOTAL WEIGHT GAIN

BELLY MEASUREMENT

BABY BUMP PHOTO

WEEKLY REFLECTIONS

SYMPTOMS & CRAVINGS

WHAT I WANT TO REMEMBER MOST

I'M MOST EXCITED ABOUT

I'M MOST NERVOUS ABOUT

Dear Baby,

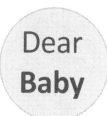

PREGNANCY *Journal*

Dear Baby

TODAY'S DATE

WEEKS PREGNANT

HOW I'M FEELING TODAY

What I want you to know

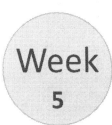

Week 5

PREGNANCY *Journal*

Your baby is the size of a peppercorn!

TOTAL WEIGHT GAIN

BELLY MEASUREMENT

BABY BUMP PHOTO

WEEKLY REFLECTIONS

SYMPTOMS & CRAVINGS

WHAT I WANT TO REMEMBER MOST

I'M MOST EXCITED ABOUT

I'M MOST NERVOUS ABOUT

Dear Baby,

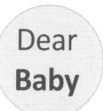

Dear
Baby

PREGNANCY *Journal*

TODAY'S DATE

WEEKS PREGNANT

HOW I'M FEELING TODAY

What I want you to know

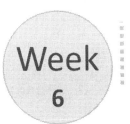

Week 6

PREGNANCY *Journal*

Your baby is the size of a sweet pea!

TOTAL WEIGHT GAIN

BELLY MEASUREMENT

BABY BUMP PHOTO

WEEKLY REFLECTIONS

SYMPTOMS & CRAVINGS

WHAT I WANT TO REMEMBER MOST

I'M MOST EXCITED ABOUT

I'M MOST NERVOUS ABOUT

Dear Baby,

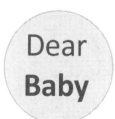

Dear Baby

PREGNANCY *Journal*

♥ ♥ ♥ ♥ ♥ ♥ ♥ ♥ ♥ ♥ ♥ ♥ ♥ ♥ ♥ ♥ ♥ ♥ ♥ ♥

TODAY'S DATE

WEEKS PREGNANT

HOW I'M FEELING TODAY

What I want you to know

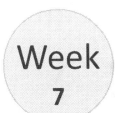

Week 7

PREGNANCY Journal

Your baby is the size of a blueberry!

TOTAL WEIGHT GAIN

BELLY MEASUREMENT

BABY BUMP PHOTO

WEEKLY REFLECTIONS

SYMPTOMS & CRAVINGS

WHAT I WANT TO REMEMBER MOST

I'M MOST EXCITED ABOUT

I'M MOST NERVOUS ABOUT

Dear Baby,

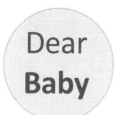

PREGNANCY *Journal*

TODAY'S DATE

WEEKS PREGNANT

HOW I'M FEELING TODAY

What I want you to know

Week 8

PREGNANCY *Journal*

Your baby is the size of a raspberry!

TOTAL WEIGHT GAIN

BELLY MEASUREMENT

BABY BUMP PHOTO

WEEKLY REFLECTIONS

SYMPTOMS & CRAVINGS

WHAT I WANT TO REMEMBER MOST

I'M MOST EXCITED ABOUT

I'M MOST NERVOUS ABOUT

Dear Baby,

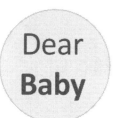

PREGNANCY *Journal*

♥ ♥ ♥ ♥ ♥ ♥ ♥ ♥ ♥ ♥ ♥ ♥ ♥ ♥ ♥ ♥ ♥ ♥

**TODAY'S
DATE**

**WEEKS
PREGNANT**

**HOW I'M
FEELING TODAY**

*What I want you to
know*

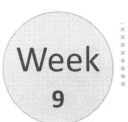

Week 9

PREGNANCY *Journal*

Your baby is the size of a grape!

TOTAL WEIGHT GAIN

BELLY MEASUREMENT

BABY BUMP PHOTO

WEEKLY REFLECTIONS

SYMPTOMS & CRAVINGS

WHAT I WANT TO REMEMBER MOST

I'M MOST EXCITED ABOUT

I'M MOST NERVOUS ABOUT

Dear Baby,

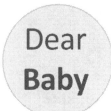

Dear Baby

PREGNANCY *Journal*

TODAY'S DATE

WEEKS PREGNANT

HOW I'M FEELING TODAY

What I want you to know

Week 10

PREGNANCY *Journal*

Your baby is the size of a prune!

TOTAL WEIGHT GAIN

BELLY MEASUREMENT

BABY BUMP PHOTO

WEEKLY REFLECTIONS

SYMPTOMS & CRAVINGS

WHAT I WANT TO REMEMBER MOST

I'M MOST EXCITED ABOUT

I'M MOST NERVOUS ABOUT

Dear Baby,

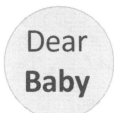

Dear Baby

PREGNANCY *Journal*

TODAY'S DATE

WEEKS PREGNANT

HOW I'M FEELING TODAY

What I want you to know

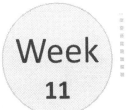

Week 11

PREGNANCY *Journal*

Your baby is the size of a lime!

TOTAL WEIGHT GAIN

BELLY MEASUREMENT

BABY BUMP PHOTO

WEEKLY REFLECTIONS

SYMPTOMS & CRAVINGS

WHAT I WANT TO REMEMBER MOST

I'M MOST EXCITED ABOUT

I'M MOST NERVOUS ABOUT

Dear Baby,

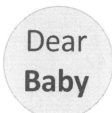

PREGNANCY *Journal*

TODAY'S DATE

WEEKS PREGNANT

HOW I'M FEELING TODAY

What I want you to know

Week 12

PREGNANCY *Journal*

Your baby is the size of a plum!

TOTAL WEIGHT GAIN

BELLY MEASUREMENT

WEEKLY REFLECTIONS

SYMPTOMS & CRAVINGS

BABY BUMP PHOTO

WHAT I WANT TO REMEMBER MOST

I'M MOST EXCITED ABOUT

I'M MOST NERVOUS ABOUT

Dear Baby,

12 WEEKS

ULTRASOUND *Scan*

ULTRASOUND PHOTO

ULTRASOUND RESULTS

BABY'S LENGTH:	
BABY'S WEIGHT:	
BPD:	
DUE DATE:	

Notes

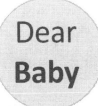

PREGNANCY *Journal*

TODAY'S DATE

WEEKS PREGNANT

HOW I'M FEELING TODAY

What I want you to know

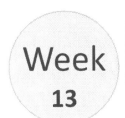

Week 13

PREGNANCY *Journal*

Your baby is the size of a peach!

TOTAL WEIGHT GAIN

BELLY MEASUREMENT

BABY BUMP PHOTO

WEEKLY REFLECTIONS

SYMPTOMS & CRAVINGS

WHAT I WANT TO REMEMBER MOST

I'M MOST EXCITED ABOUT

I'M MOST NERVOUS ABOUT

Dear Baby,

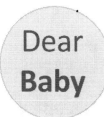

Dear Baby

PREGNANCY *Journal*

TODAY'S DATE

WEEKS PREGNANT

HOW I'M FEELING TODAY

What I want you to know

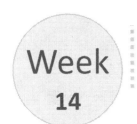

Week 14

PREGNANCY *Journal*

Your baby is the size of a lemon!

TOTAL WEIGHT GAIN

BELLY MEASUREMENT

BABY BUMP PHOTO

WEEKLY REFLECTIONS

SYMPTOMS & CRAVINGS

WHAT I WANT TO REMEMBER MOST

I'M MOST EXCITED ABOUT

I'M MOST NERVOUS ABOUT

Dear Baby,

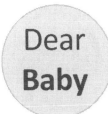

PREGNANCY *Journal*

TODAY'S DATE

WEEKS PREGNANT

HOW I'M FEELING TODAY

What I want you to know

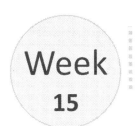

Week 15

PREGNANCY *Journal*

Your baby is the size of an apple!

TOTAL WEIGHT GAIN

BELLY MEASUREMENT

BABY BUMP PHOTO

WEEKLY REFLECTIONS

SYMPTOMS & CRAVINGS

WHAT I WANT TO REMEMBER MOST

I'M MOST EXCITED ABOUT

I'M MOST NERVOUS ABOUT

Dear Baby,

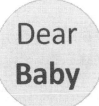

PREGNANCY *Journal*

TODAY'S DATE

WEEKS PREGNANT

HOW I'M FEELING TODAY

What I want you to know

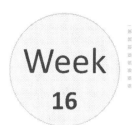

Week 16

PREGNANCY *Journal*

Your baby is the size of an avocado!

TOTAL WEIGHT GAIN

BELLY MEASUREMENT

BABY BUMP PHOTO

WEEKLY REFLECTIONS

SYMPTOMS & CRAVINGS

WHAT I WANT TO REMEMBER MOST

I'M MOST EXCITED ABOUT

I'M MOST NERVOUS ABOUT

Dear Baby,

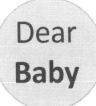

PREGNANCY *Journal*

TODAY'S DATE

WEEKS PREGNANT

HOW I'M FEELING TODAY

What I want you to know

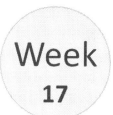

Week 17

PREGNANCY *Journal*

Your baby is the size of a pear!

TOTAL WEIGHT GAIN

BELLY MEASUREMENT

BABY BUMP PHOTO

WEEKLY REFLECTIONS

SYMPTOMS & CRAVINGS

WHAT I WANT TO REMEMBER MOST

I'M MOST EXCITED ABOUT

I'M MOST NERVOUS ABOUT

Dear Baby,

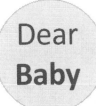

PREGNANCY *Journal*

TODAY'S DATE

WEEKS PREGNANT

HOW I'M FEELING TODAY

What I want you to know

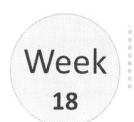

Week 18

PREGNANCY *Journal*

Your baby is the size of a sweet potato!

TOTAL WEIGHT GAIN

BELLY MEASUREMENT

BABY BUMP PHOTO

WEEKLY REFLECTIONS

SYMPTOMS & CRAVINGS

WHAT I WANT TO REMEMBER MOST

I'M MOST EXCITED ABOUT

I'M MOST NERVOUS ABOUT

Dear Baby,

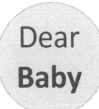

PREGNANCY *Journal*

TODAY'S DATE

WEEKS PREGNANT

HOW I'M FEELING TODAY

What I want you to know

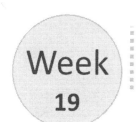

Week 19

PREGNANCY Journal

Your baby is the size of a mango!

TOTAL WEIGHT GAIN

BELLY MEASUREMENT

BABY BUMP PHOTO

WEEKLY REFLECTIONS

SYMPTOMS & CRAVINGS

WHAT I WANT TO REMEMBER MOST

I'M MOST EXCITED ABOUT

I'M MOST NERVOUS ABOUT

Dear Baby,

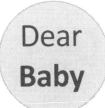

Dear Baby

PREGNANCY *Journal*

TODAY'S DATE

WEEKS PREGNANT

HOW I'M FEELING TODAY

What I want you to know

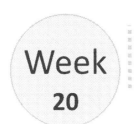

Week 20

PREGNANCY *Journal*

Your baby is the size of a banana!

TOTAL WEIGHT GAIN

BELLY MEASUREMENT

BABY BUMP PHOTO

WEEKLY REFLECTIONS

SYMPTOMS & CRAVINGS

WHAT I WANT TO REMEMBER MOST

I'M MOST EXCITED ABOUT

I'M MOST NERVOUS ABOUT

Dear Baby,

20 WEEKS

ULTRASOUND *Scan*

ULTRASOUND PHOTO

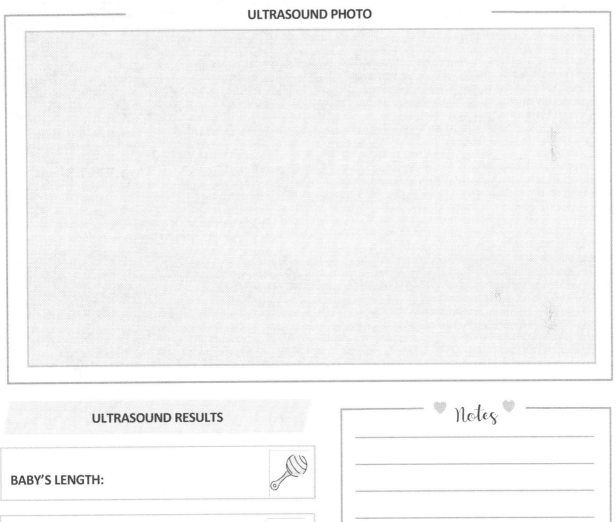

ULTRASOUND RESULTS

BABY'S LENGTH:

BABY'S WEIGHT:

BPD:

DUE DATE:

Notes

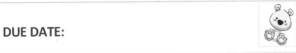

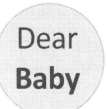

PREGNANCY *Journal*

TODAY'S DATE

WEEKS PREGNANT

HOW I'M FEELING TODAY

What I want you to know

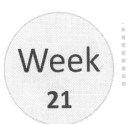

Week 21

PREGNANCY *Journal*

Your baby is the size of a carrot!

TOTAL WEIGHT GAIN	BELLY MEASUREMENT

WEEKLY REFLECTIONS

SYMPTOMS & CRAVINGS

BABY BUMP PHOTO

WHAT I WANT TO REMEMBER MOST

I'M MOST EXCITED ABOUT

I'M MOST NERVOUS ABOUT

Dear Baby,

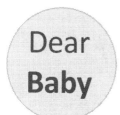

Dear Baby

PREGNANCY *Journal*

♥ ♥ ♥ ♥ ♥ ♥ ♥ ♥ ♥ ♥ ♥ ♥ ♥ ♥ ♥ ♥ ♥ ♥ ♥ ♥

TODAY'S DATE

WEEKS PREGNANT

HOW I'M FEELING TODAY

What I want you to know

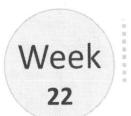

Week 22

PREGNANCY *Journal*

Your baby is the size of a papaya!

TOTAL WEIGHT GAIN

BELLY MEASUREMENT

BABY BUMP PHOTO

WEEKLY REFLECTIONS

SYMPTOMS & CRAVINGS

WHAT I WANT TO REMEMBER MOST

I'M MOST EXCITED ABOUT

I'M MOST NERVOUS ABOUT

Dear Baby,

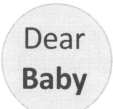

Dear Baby

PREGNANCY *Journal*

TODAY'S DATE

WEEKS PREGNANT

HOW I'M FEELING TODAY

What I want you to know

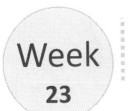

Week 23

PREGNANCY *Journal*

Your baby is the size of a grapefruit!

TOTAL WEIGHT GAIN

BELLY MEASUREMENT

BABY BUMP PHOTO

WEEKLY REFLECTIONS

SYMPTOMS & CRAVINGS

WHAT I WANT TO REMEMBER MOST

I'M MOST EXCITED ABOUT

I'M MOST NERVOUS ABOUT

Dear Baby,

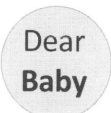

Dear Baby

PREGNANCY *Journal*

TODAY'S DATE

WEEKS PREGNANT

HOW I'M FEELING TODAY

What I want you to know

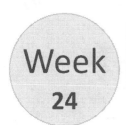

Week 24

PREGNANCY *Journal*

Your baby is the size of a cantaloupe!

TOTAL WEIGHT GAIN

BELLY MEASUREMENT

BABY BUMP PHOTO

WEEKLY REFLECTIONS

SYMPTOMS & CRAVINGS

WHAT I WANT TO REMEMBER MOST

I'M MOST EXCITED ABOUT

I'M MOST NERVOUS ABOUT

Dear Baby,

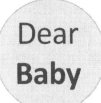

Dear Baby

PREGNANCY *Journal*

TODAY'S DATE

WEEKS PREGNANT

HOW I'M FEELING TODAY

What I want you to know

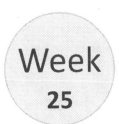

Week 25

PREGNANCY *Journal*

Your baby is the size of a cauliflower!

TOTAL WEIGHT GAIN

BELLY MEASUREMENT

BABY BUMP PHOTO

WEEKLY REFLECTIONS

SYMPTOMS & CRAVINGS

WHAT I WANT TO REMEMBER MOST

I'M MOST EXCITED ABOUT

I'M MOST NERVOUS ABOUT

Dear Baby,

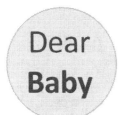

PREGNANCY *Journal*

TODAY'S DATE

WEEKS PREGNANT

HOW I'M FEELING TODAY

What I want you to know

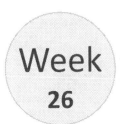

Week 26

PREGNANCY *Journal*

Your baby is the size of a head of lettuce!

TOTAL WEIGHT GAIN

BELLY MEASUREMENT

BABY BUMP PHOTO

WEEKLY REFLECTIONS

SYMPTOMS & CRAVINGS

WHAT I WANT TO REMEMBER MOST

I'M MOST EXCITED ABOUT

I'M MOST NERVOUS ABOUT

Dear Baby,

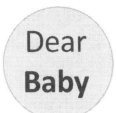

Dear Baby

PREGNANCY *Journal*

♥ ♥ ♥ ♥ ♥ ♥ ♥ ♥ ♥ ♥ ♥ ♥ ♥ ♥ ♥ ♥ ♥ ♥ ♥ ♥

TODAY'S DATE

WEEKS PREGNANT

HOW I'M FEELING TODAY

What I want you to know

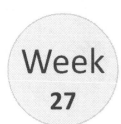

Week 27

PREGNANCY *Journal*

Your baby is the size of a rutabaga!

TOTAL WEIGHT GAIN

BELLY MEASUREMENT

BABY BUMP PHOTO

WEEKLY REFLECTIONS

SYMPTOMS & CRAVINGS

WHAT I WANT TO REMEMBER MOST

I'M MOST EXCITED ABOUT

I'M MOST NERVOUS ABOUT

Dear Baby,

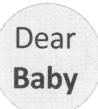

Dear Baby

PREGNANCY *Journal*

TODAY'S DATE

WEEKS PREGNANT

HOW I'M FEELING TODAY

What I want you to know

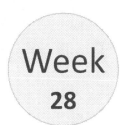

Week 28

PREGNANCY *Journal*

Your baby is the size of an eggplant!

TOTAL WEIGHT GAIN

BELLY MEASUREMENT

BABY BUMP PHOTO

WEEKLY REFLECTIONS

SYMPTOMS & CRAVINGS

WHAT I WANT TO REMEMBER MOST

I'M MOST EXCITED ABOUT

I'M MOST NERVOUS ABOUT

Dear Baby,

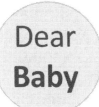

Dear Baby

PREGNANCY *Journal*

♥♥♥♥♥♥♥♥♥♥♥♥♥♥♥♥♥♥♥♥♥♥♥♥

TODAY'S DATE

WEEKS PREGNANT

HOW I'M FEELING TODAY

What I want you to know

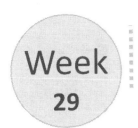

Week 29

PREGNANCY *Journal*

Your baby is the size of an acorn squash!

TOTAL WEIGHT GAIN

BELLY MEASUREMENT

BABY BUMP PHOTO

WEEKLY REFLECTIONS

SYMPTOMS & CRAVINGS

WHAT I WANT TO REMEMBER MOST

I'M MOST EXCITED ABOUT

I'M MOST NERVOUS ABOUT

Dear Baby,

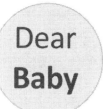

Dear Baby

PREGNANCY *Journal*

TODAY'S DATE

WEEKS PREGNANT

HOW I'M FEELING TODAY

What I want you to know

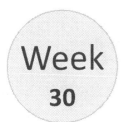

Week 30

PREGNANCY *Journal*

Your baby is the size of a cucumber!

TOTAL WEIGHT GAIN

BELLY MEASUREMENT

BABY BUMP PHOTO

WEEKLY REFLECTIONS

SYMPTOMS & CRAVINGS

WHAT I WANT TO REMEMBER MOST

I'M MOST EXCITED ABOUT

I'M MOST NERVOUS ABOUT

Dear Baby,

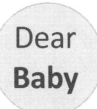

Dear Baby

PREGNANCY *Journal*

TODAY'S DATE

WEEKS PREGNANT

HOW I'M FEELING TODAY

What I want you to know

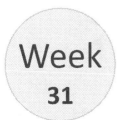

Week 31

PREGNANCY *Journal*

Your baby is the size of a pineapple!

TOTAL WEIGHT GAIN

BELLY MEASUREMENT

BABY BUMP PHOTO

WEEKLY REFLECTIONS

SYMPTOMS & CRAVINGS

WHAT I WANT TO REMEMBER MOST

I'M MOST EXCITED ABOUT

I'M MOST NERVOUS ABOUT

Dear Baby,

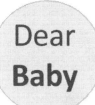

Dear Baby

PREGNANCY *Journal*

TODAY'S DATE

WEEKS PREGNANT

HOW I'M FEELING TODAY

What I want you to know

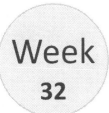

Week 32

PREGNANCY *Journal*

Your baby is the size of a squash!

TOTAL WEIGHT GAIN

BELLY MEASUREMENT

BABY BUMP PHOTO

WEEKLY REFLECTIONS

SYMPTOMS & CRAVINGS

WHAT I WANT TO REMEMBER MOST

I'M MOST EXCITED ABOUT

I'M MOST NERVOUS ABOUT

Dear Baby,

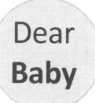

PREGNANCY *Journal*

TODAY'S DATE

WEEKS PREGNANT

HOW I'M FEELING TODAY

What I want you to know

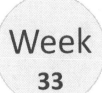

Week 33

PREGNANCY *Journal*

Your baby is the size of a durian!

TOTAL WEIGHT GAIN

BELLY MEASUREMENT

BABY BUMP PHOTO

WEEKLY REFLECTIONS

SYMPTOMS & CRAVINGS

WHAT I WANT TO REMEMBER MOST

I'M MOST EXCITED ABOUT

I'M MOST NERVOUS ABOUT

Dear Baby,

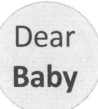

Dear Baby

PREGNANCY *Journal*

♥♥♥♥♥♥♥♥♥♥♥♥♥♥♥♥♥♥♥♥

TODAY'S DATE

WEEKS PREGNANT

HOW I'M FEELING TODAY

What I want you to know

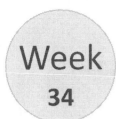

Week 34

PREGNANCY *Journal*

Your baby is the size of a butternut squash!

TOTAL WEIGHT GAIN

BELLY MEASUREMENT

BABY BUMP PHOTO

WEEKLY REFLECTIONS

SYMPTOMS & CRAVINGS

WHAT I WANT TO REMEMBER MOST

I'M MOST EXCITED ABOUT

I'M MOST NERVOUS ABOUT

Dear Baby,

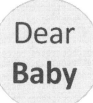

Dear Baby

PREGNANCY *Journal*

♥♥♥♥♥♥♥♥♥♥♥♥♥♥♥♥♥♥♥♥♥♥

TODAY'S DATE

WEEKS PREGNANT

HOW I'M FEELING TODAY

What I want you to know

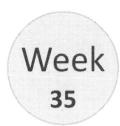

Week 35

PREGNANCY *Journal*

Your baby is the size of a coconut!

TOTAL WEIGHT GAIN

BELLY MEASUREMENT

WEEKLY REFLECTIONS

SYMPTOMS & CRAVINGS

BABY BUMP PHOTO

WHAT I WANT TO REMEMBER MOST

I'M MOST EXCITED ABOUT

I'M MOST NERVOUS ABOUT

Dear Baby,

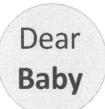

PREGNANCY *Journal*

TODAY'S DATE

WEEKS PREGNANT

HOW I'M FEELING TODAY

What I want you to know

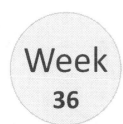

Week 36

PREGNANCY *Journal*

Your baby is the size of a honeydew melon!

TOTAL WEIGHT GAIN

BELLY MEASUREMENT

BABY BUMP PHOTO

WEEKLY REFLECTIONS

SYMPTOMS & CRAVINGS

WHAT I WANT TO REMEMBER MOST

I'M MOST EXCITED ABOUT

I'M MOST NERVOUS ABOUT

Dear Baby,

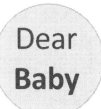

Dear
Baby

PREGNANCY *Journal*

♥♥♥♥♥♥♥♥♥♥♥♥♥♥♥♥♥♥♥♥♥♥♥♥

**TODAY'S
DATE**

**WEEKS
PREGNANT**

**HOW I'M
FEELING TODAY**

*What I want you to
know*

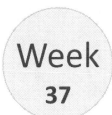

Week 37

PREGNANCY *Journal*

Your baby is the size of a Winter Melon!

TOTAL WEIGHT GAIN

BELLY MEASUREMENT

BABY BUMP PHOTO

WEEKLY REFLECTIONS

SYMPTOMS & CRAVINGS

WHAT I WANT TO REMEMBER MOST

I'M MOST EXCITED ABOUT

I'M MOST NERVOUS ABOUT

Dear Baby,

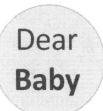

Dear Baby

PREGNANCY *Journal*

TODAY'S DATE

WEEKS PREGNANT

HOW I'M FEELING TODAY

What I want you to know

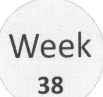

Week 38

PREGNANCY *Journal*

Your baby is the size of a pumpkin!

TOTAL WEIGHT GAIN

BELLY MEASUREMENT

BABY BUMP PHOTO

WEEKLY REFLECTIONS

SYMPTOMS & CRAVINGS

WHAT I WANT TO REMEMBER MOST

I'M MOST EXCITED ABOUT

I'M MOST NERVOUS ABOUT

Dear Baby,

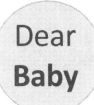

Dear Baby

PREGNANCY *Journal*

TODAY'S DATE

WEEKS PREGNANT

HOW I'M FEELING TODAY

What I want you to know

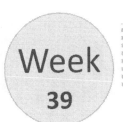

Week 39

PREGNANCY *Journal*

Your baby is the size of a watermelon!

TOTAL WEIGHT GAIN	BELLY MEASUREMENT

WEEKLY REFLECTIONS

_____
_____
_____
_____
_____
_____
_____

SYMPTOMS & CRAVINGS

_____
_____
_____
_____

BABY BUMP PHOTO

WHAT I WANT TO REMEMBER MOST

I'M MOST EXCITED ABOUT

I'M MOST NERVOUS ABOUT

Dear Baby,

_____
_____
_____
_____
_____
_____
_____
_____
_____
_____
_____

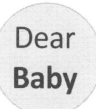

PREGNANCY *Journal*

TODAY'S DATE

WEEKS PREGNANT

HOW I'M FEELING TODAY

What I want you to know

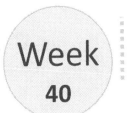

Week 40

PREGNANCY *Journal*

Your baby is the size of a jack fruit!

TOTAL WEIGHT GAIN

BELLY MEASUREMENT

BABY BUMP PHOTO

WEEKLY REFLECTIONS

SYMPTOMS & CRAVINGS

WHAT I WANT TO REMEMBER MOST

I'M MOST EXCITED ABOUT

I'M MOST NERVOUS ABOUT

Dear Baby,

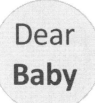

PREGNANCY *Journal*

TODAY'S DATE

WEEKS PREGNANT

HOW I'M FEELING TODAY

What I want you to know

Made in the USA
Middletown, DE
26 November 2023

43618805R00057